YOUR KNOWLEDGE HAS VALUE

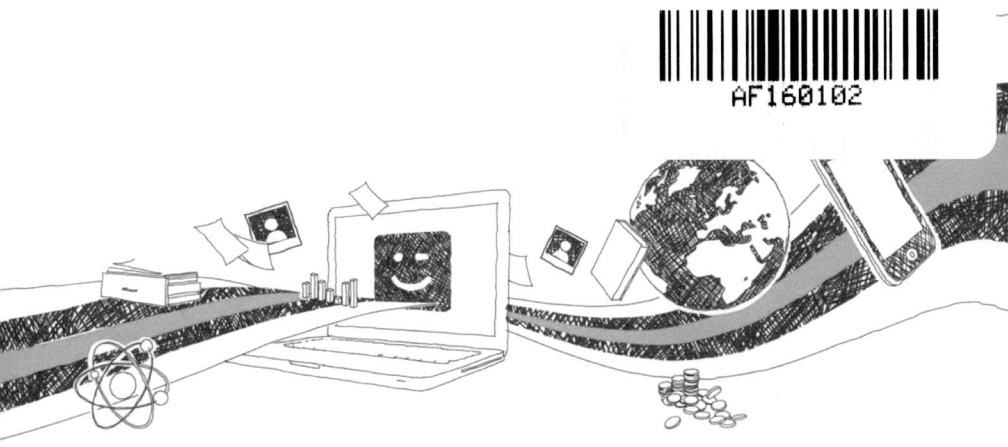

- We will publish your bachelor's and master's thesis, essays and papers

- Your own eBook and book - sold worldwide in all relevant shops

- Earn money with each sale

Upload your text at www.GRIN.com and publish for free

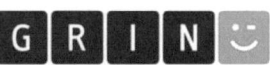

Bibliographic information published by the German National Library:

The German National Library lists this publication in the National Bibliography; detailed bibliographic data are available on the Internet at http://dnb.dnb.de .

This book is copyright material and must not be copied, reproduced, transferred, distributed, leased, licensed or publicly performed or used in any way except as specifically permitted in writing by the publishers, as allowed under the terms and conditions under which it was purchased or as strictly permitted by applicable copyright law. Any unauthorized distribution or use of this text may be a direct infringement of the author s and publisher s rights and those responsible may be liable in law accordingly.

Imprint:

Copyright © 2017 GRIN Verlag, Open Publishing GmbH
Print and binding: Books on Demand GmbH, Norderstedt Germany
ISBN: 9783668584747

This book at GRIN:

http://www.grin.com/en/e-book/380718/the-revelance-of-homeopathy-in-pregnancy-childbirth-and-parturition

Patrick Kimuyu

The revelance of homeopathy in pregnancy, childbirth and parturition

GRIN Publishing

GRIN - Your knowledge has value

Since its foundation in 1998, GRIN has specialized in publishing academic texts by students, college teachers and other academics as e-book and printed book. The website www.grin.com is an ideal platform for presenting term papers, final papers, scientific essays, dissertations and specialist books.

Visit us on the internet:

http://www.grin.com/

http://www.facebook.com/grincom

http://www.twitter.com/grin_com

HOMEOPATHY FOR PREGNANCY AND DELIVERY

Author: Patrick K. Kimuyu

Inhaltsverzeichnis

Introduction 3

Conditions during Pregnancy and Delivery 4

Role of Homeopathic Medicines during Pregnancy 5

Homeopathic Medicines for Morning Sickness 5

Homeopathic Medicines for Breech Birth 6

Role of Homeopathic Medicines in Post-Delivery Processes 7

Conclusion 8

References 9

Introduction

Pregnancy and childbirth phenomena are considered to be among the most fundamental issues in one's life. These are the early stages of life and, they seem to be delicate and difficult to manage. However, the field of medicine has grown extensively to accommodate all the possible challenges associated with pregnancy and delivery. Currently, there are a number of sophisticated medical procedures, which appear to have eliminated pain and increased the safety of the mother and child. In the past, pregnancy and delivery were some of the most painful ordeals to women and, could result into death at times, owing to pregnancy complications (Hershoff, 2000). Ordinarily, the fetus developmental process is accompanied by diverse biological changes in the fetus and the pregnant mother, as well. Some of the developmental changes cause biochemical interferences to the normal biological functioning of the body, leading to the observed conditions during pregnancy. On the other hand, pregnancy and childbirth are accompanied with a number of fatalities; thus, healthcare professionals have seemingly become victims of circumstance, in case there are fatal outcomes. As a result, healthcare professionals in public and private healthcare facilities are currently administering heavy drug doses to pregnant mothers, especially during delivery to hasten labor and suppress pain. However, they have adopted this new approach to evade lawsuits related to the medical ethics, in case they perform delivery with fatal outcome. Alternatively, homeopathy has currently emerged as the most appropriate approach towards addressing the enormous health challenges associated with conventional medical procedures. Therefore, this research will give an overview of homeopathy and its relevance in pregnancy, childbirth and after parturition.

Conditions during Pregnancy and Delivery

It is evidently true that pregnancy is a lengthy process with numerous biological changes. It begins with conception, which is relatively a simple biological process. However, other stages of fetal development, which follow after conception up to the post-parturition process, are quite delicate and, they encompass transient biochemical reactions. One of the most remarkable biological processes, which occur during pregnancy, is the morning sickness, which is quite unpleasant to most pregnant mothers (Hershoff, 2000). Ordinarily, morning sickness occurs towards the end of the first trimester during a maternal process referred to as 'selfing', when the maternal body recognizes the fetus as 'self'. Therefore, biological conditions experienced during morning sickness are attributable to the biological changes in the fetal and the maternal body systems.

From a medical perspective, homeopathy becomes relevant from this first process of the fetal development and, it has been found to be useful, even after child delivery. Some of the most fundamental processes where homeopathy has been found helpful include the entire process of pregnancy, parturition and post-delivery processes. In general, there are series of processes involved and, each of these has appropriate homeopathic medicines, which can be administered to address the involved health conditions. Surprisingly, homeopathic remedies are believed to be quite useful during pregnancy complications. Some of the processes, in which homeopathy aids include morning sickness, breech birth, labor, retained placenta and post-partum hemorrhage. It has also been found to be useful in asphyxia of newborn, post-natal depression and perineal episiotomies (Schmukler, 2003). Moreover, homeopathy offers alternative medicines for facilitating healing after birth and breastfeeding.

Role of Homeopathic Medicines during Pregnancy

Homeopathic medicines are used to solve different biological processes during pregnancy. Some of the medicines are useful in one area, whereas others are universal. The usefulness of these medicines can be explained by the roles they play during episodes of morning sickness, breech birth and labor.

Homeopathic Medicines for Morning Sickness

Morning sickness is usually a normal biological process but, not a sickness; although its manifestations are, more or less similar to those of some disease conditions. Nausea is believed to be one of the most popular signs of morning sickness. Others include mood swings, allergic reactions from the surrounding environment, vomiting, diarrhea and polyphagia. Episodes of loss of sleep are also experienced by pregnant women, especially during the early stages of pregnancy (Schmukler, 2003). These conditions can be relieved with homeopathic remedies for pleasant healthy feeling during pregnancy.

Some of the homeopathic medicines, which are useful in relieving the effects of morning sickness, include Anacardium, Cocculus, Colchicum, Pulsatilla, Veratrum alb and Symphoricarpus. Anacardium relieves nausea and vomiting, whereas Cocculus and Pulsatilla relieve excessive salivation and mood swings respectively. Symphoricarpus and Veratrum alb are useful remedies for constipation and vomiting with diarrhea (Tayler, 2007).

However, it is worth noting that the symptoms, upon which these medicines are administered, are relatively different. For instance, Anacardium, Nux Vomica, Ipecac, Symphoricarpus and Pulsatilla are reliable remedies for morning sickness, especially when the woman is experiencing nausea conditions but, the nature of the condition determines the most appropriate medicines to be administered to the pregnant woman. Pulsatilla is usually suitable for pregnant women weepy and needy, whereas Nux Vomica is preferable for pregnant women who display anger and irritability (Hugall, 2004).

In regard to the nature of the nausea, Anacardium is administered to pregnant women whose nausea is relieved by ingestion of food, whereas, Ipecac and Symphoricarpus are preferable for pregnant women whose nausea is continuous and deathly. Ipecac is usually helpful to pregnant women who experience continuous nausea, which does not subside after vomiting. In contrast, Symphoricarpus is preferable to constipated pregnant women with continuous vomiting and episodes of retching (Hugall, 2004).

Homeopathic Medicines for Breech Birth

Breech birth is a condition in which the fetus does not assume the ordinary birth position of head first towards the end of the third trimester of pregnancy (Schmukler, 2003). Natrum Muriaticum and Pulsatilla remedies are known to facilitate the positioning of the fetus before birth. These remedies are known to move the fetus from the breech position within a short duration by stimulating the activity of the uterine muscles. However, it is worth noting that, these medicines do not function in the same way, even though they address common problems.

Natrum Muriaticum is usually used when the mother is experiencing loneliness and, she portrays emotional feelings. These symptoms can be identified when the mother tends to remain alone, crying for no apparent reason known to the homeopath (Hugall, 2004).

In contrast, Pulsatilla is usually used when the mother tends to be highly sympathetic and in need of company. In such situations, the mother craves for fresh air, displaying tendencies of crying and weeping. Therefore, the symptoms, which require Pulsatilla are completely opposite to those requiring Natrum Muriaticum (Hugall, 2004).

Homeopathic Medicines and Labor

Labor is an extensive biological process, which involves intensive contraction of uterine muscles under the effect of Oxytocin and prostaglandins such as PGF2α. This process is usually accompanied by intense pain; therefore, homeopathic medicines such as Caulophyllum, Aconite and Chamomilla help to relieve pain, resulting from painful uterine contractions.

Caulophyllum is administered to pregnant women who tend to be restless and nervous, with irregular labor pains. These women desire company but, they are hardly talkative because; claim to experience severe pain in the entire body (Hugall, 2004).

On the other hand, Chamomilla is applied to aid women with painful contractions, who usually express anger, resulting from labor pains. Such women are irritable and abusive; thus, they are difficult to control (Hugall, 2004).

In addition, Pulsatilla can be administered to the woman in labor to initiate the parturition process (Castro, 2005).

Role of Homeopathic Medicines in Post-Delivery Processes

In most cases, parturition is followed by a number of complications such as retained placenta, post-partum bleeding, post-natal depression and asphyxia of the newborn and, homeopathic medicines have proven to be useful. For instance, Syntometrine, Pulsatilla and Cantharis remedies aid in enhancing uterine muscles contraction to expel the placenta (Schmukler, 2003).

On the other hand, the separation of the umbilical cord and the placenta may cause stress on the endometrial walls, resulting into post-partum hemorrhage. Excessive bleeding is prevented with the administration of Cinchona (Tayler, 2007). Post-natal depression is usually alleviated by the use of Platina, Natrum Muriaticum and Aconite. Aconite relieves panic, especially when the mother experiences post-partum bleeding. Moreover, there are homeopathic medicines for healing of perineal tears and episiotomies (Hugall, 2004). Some of the most useful remedies are Calendula, Hypericum and Arnica (Castro, 2005). These remedies are known to control swelling and bleeding of torn tissues and, Arnica prevents pathogenic infections due to its antimicrobial potency. In addition, Carbo veg enable newborns that experience Oxygen deficiency to recover efficiently without incidences of jaundice (Gaskin, 2011).

Conclusion

In a brief conclusion, homeopathy serves as a reliable medical approach, which does not encompass breach to the medical legal ethics. It has emerged to be a live-saving approach because; it addresses numerous pregnancy complications. Moreover, it is highly reliable because; there are no sophisticated medical equipments are required; instead, the process requires an extensive knowledge on the homeopathic remedies to administer in different situations and dosage. It is also worth noting that, homeopathy plays a pivotal role in reducing the use of conventional medicines; thus, alleviating their side-effects. Therefore, homeopathy is highly recommended as the only remedy to fatalities encountered in the conventional medical profession.

References

Castro, M. (2005). *Homeopathy for Mother and Baby: Pregnancy, Birth and the Post Natal Year*. Norfolk, UK: Homoeopathic Supply Co.

Gaskin, I. (2011). *Birth Matters: A Midwife's Manifesta*. London, UK: Pinter & Martin Ltd.

Hershoff, A. (2000). *Homeopathic Remedies: A Quick and Easy Guide to Common Disorders and Their Homeopathic Remedies*. New York, NY: Penguin Group.

Hugall, L. (2004). *Pregnancy & Childbirth Made Easier with Homeopathy*. http://hpathy.com/homeopathy-papers/pregnancy-childbirth-made-easier-with-homeopathy/

Schmukler, A. (2003). *Homeopathy: The Home Handbook for Survival*. Bloomington, In: Xlibris Corporation.

Tayler, R. (2007). *Homeopathy for Pregnancy and Childbirth*. Ottawa, ON: Ottawa School of Homeopathy.

YOUR KNOWLEDGE HAS VALUE

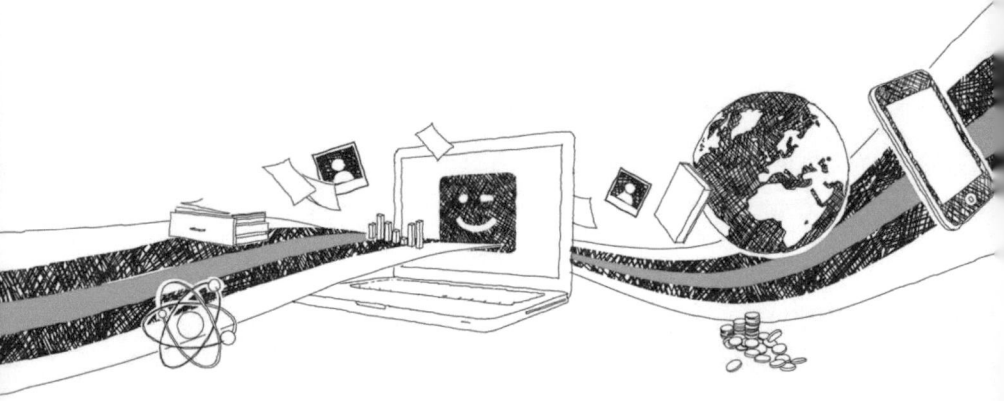

- We will publish your bachelor's and master's thesis, essays and papers

- Your own eBook and book - sold worldwide in all relevant shops

- Earn money with each sale

Upload your text at www.GRIN.com
and publish for free

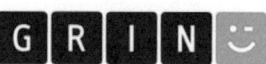